Contents

Cannabis Extract

Introduction

Cannabis is a natural product, the main psychoactive constituent of which is tetrahydrocannabinol ($\Delta 9$-THC). The cannabis plant (Cannabis sativa L.) is broadly distributed and grows in temperate and tropical areas. Together with tobacco, alcohol and caffeine, it is one of the most widely consumed drugs throughout the world, and has been used as a drug and a source of fibre since historical times. Herbal cannabis consists of the dried flowering tops and leaves. Cannabis resin is a compressed solid made from the resinous parts of the plant, and cannabis (hash) oil is a solvent extract of cannabis. Cannabis is almost always smoked, often mixed with tobacco. Almost all consumption of herbal cannabis and resin is of illicit material. Some therapeutic benefit as an analgesic has been claimed for cannabis, and dronabinol is a licensed medicine in some countries for the treatment of nausea in cancer chemotherapy. Cannabis products and Δ9-THC are under international control.

Chemistry

The major active principle in all cannabis products is Δ9- tetrahydrocannabinol (Δ9-THC or simply THC), also known by its International Non-Proprietary Name (INN) as dronabinol. The unsaturated bond in the cyclohexene ring is located between C-9 and C-10 in the more common dibenzopyran ring numbering system. There are four stereoisomers of THC, but only the (–)-trans isomer occurs naturally (CAS-1972-08-03). The fully systematic name for this THC isomer is (–)-(6aR,10aR)-6,6,9-trimethyl-3-pentyl- 6a,7,8,10a-tetrahydro-6H-benzo[c]chromen-1-ol. Two related substances, Δ9- tetrahydrocannabinol-2-oic acid and Δ9-tetrahydrocannabinol-4-oic acid (THCA), are also present in cannabis, sometimes in large amounts. During smoking, THCA is partly converted to THC.

The active isomer Δ8-THC, in which the unsaturated bond in the cyclohexene ring is located between C-8 and C-9, is found in much smaller amounts.

Molecular structure (1)

Other closely related substances that occur in cannabis include cannabidiol (CBD) and, in aged samples, cannabinol (CBN), both of which have quite different pharmacological effects to THC. Other compounds include the cannabivarins and cannabichromenes; they are all collectively known as cannabinoids. Unlike many psychoactive substances, cannabinoids are not nitrogenous bases.

(1) Δ9-tetrahydrocannabinol, the major psychoactive principle of cannabis, showing the partial ring numbering system in the more common dibenzofuran system.

Physical form

Cannabis sativa is dioecious: there are separate male and female plants. The THC is largely concentrated around the flowering parts of the female plant. The leaves and male plants have less THC, while the stalks and seeds contain almost none. Plants have characteristic compound leaves with up to 11 separate serrated lobes. Imported herbal cannabis occurs as compressed blocks of dried brown vegetable matter comprising the flowering tops, leaves, stalks and seeds of Cannabis sativa. Cannabis resin is usually produced in 250-g blocks, many of which carry a brandmark impression. Cannabis oil is a dark viscous liquid.

Pharmacology

The pharmacology of cannabis is complicated by the presence of a wide range of cannabinoids. At small doses, cannabis produces euphoria, relief of anxiety, sedation and drowsiness. In some respects, the effects are similar to those caused by alcohol. Anandamide has been identified as the endogenous ligand for the cannabinoid receptor and has pharmacological properties similar to those of THC. When cannabis is smoked, THC can be detected in plasma within seconds of inhalation; it has a half-life of 2 hours. Following smoking of the equivalent of 10–15 mg over a period of 5–7 minutes, peak plasma levels of $\Delta 9$-THC are around 100 µg/L. It is highly lipophilic and widely distributed in the body. Two active metabolites are formed: 11-hydroxy-$\Delta 9$-THC and 8β-hydroxy-$\Delta 9$-THC. The first is further metabolised to $\Delta 9$-THC-11-oic acid. Two inactive substances are also formed — 8α-hydroxy-$\Delta 9$-THC and 8α,11-dihydroxy-$\Delta 9$-THC — and many other minor metabolites, most of which appear in the urine and faeces as glucuronide conjugates. Some metabolites can be detected in the urine for up to 2 weeks following smoking or ingestion. There is little evidence for damage to organ systems among moderate users, but consumption with tobacco carries all of the risks of that substance. Most interest in the adverse properties of cannabis has centred on its association with schizophrenia, although it is still unclear if there is a causative relation between mental health and cannabis. Fatalities directly attributable to cannabis are rare.

Origin

Herbal cannabis imported into Europe may originate from West Africa, the Caribbean or South-East Asia, but cannabis resin derives largely from either North Africa or Afghanistan. Cannabis oil (hash oil) is often produced locally from cannabis or cannabis resin by means of solvent extraction. Intensive indoor cultivation has become widespread in Europe and elsewhere. This is based on improved seed varieties and procedures such as artificial heating and lighting, hydroponic cultivation in nutrient solutions and propagation of cuttings of female plants. It leads to a high production of flowering material (sometimes known as 'skunk'). As with other naturally occurring drugs of misuse (e.g. heroin and cocaine), total synthesis is not currently an economic proposition. No precursors to THC are listed in the United Nations 1988 Convention against Illicit Traffic in Narcotic Drugs and Psychotropic Substances.

Mode of use

Cannabis is usually smoked, often mixed with tobacco or in a smoking device (bong). Because THC has a low water solubility, ingestion of cannabis leads to poor absorption. The average 'reefer' cigarette contains around 200 mg of herbal cannabis or cannabis resin.

Other names

In many countries, herbal cannabis and cannabis resin are formally known as marijuana and hashish (or just 'hash') respectively. Cannabis cigarettes may be termed reefers, joints or spliffs.Street terms for cannabis/cannabis resin include bhang, charas, pot, dope, ganja, hemp, weed, blow, grass and many others.

Analysis

Although the leaves of Cannabis sativa are reasonably characteristic, cannabis and cannabis resin can both be positively identified by low-power microscopy, where the appearance of glandular trichomes and cystolithic hairs is diagnostic. The Duquenois test is considered to be specific for cannabinols. It is based on the reaction of cannabis extracts with p-dimethylbenzaldehyde. This produces a violet blue coloration that is extractable into chloroform. The mass spectrum of THC shows major ions at m/z = 299, 231, 314, 43, 41, 295, 55 and 271. Using gas chromatography, the limit of detection of THC in blood is 0.3 µg/L.

Cannabis and cannabis resin are listed in Schedules I and IV of the United Nations 1961 Single Convention on Narcotic Drugs. In Article 1, Paragraph 1, of that Convention, cannabis is defined as: 'The flowering or fruiting tops of the cannabis plant (excluding the seeds and leaves when not accompanied by the tops) from which the resin has not been extracted, by whatever name they may be designated.' Cannabis resin is defined as: 'The separated resin, whether crude or purified, obtained from the cannabis plant.' Along with a number of its isomers and stereochemical variants, $\Delta 9$-THC is listed in Schedule I of the United Nations 1971 Convention on Psychotropic Substances.

Medical use

Tinctures of cannabis (ethanolic extracts) were once common, but were removed from pharmacopoeias many years ago. Herbal cannabis (known as 'cannabis flos'), with a nominal THC content of 18 %, is available as a prescription medicine in The Netherlands. It is indicated for multiple sclerosis, certain types of pain and other neurological conditions. An extract of cannabis (Sativex) has been licensed in Canada.

Cannabis has been a part of human history for a millennium. Until the early 20th century, it was used as medicine and a spiritual guide in cultures all over the planet.

In the early 1900's it was possible to purchase cannabis tincture at pharmacies, but soon the United States federal government launched a crusade to prohibit this most intriguing plant.

For the last 80 years or so, the major drivers of medical research, pharmaceutical companies, have focused on profitable synthetic drugs and little research has been done on cannabis chemistry and therapeutic applications.

While cannabinoids like THC and CBD are well known and often thought of as the active ingredients in cannabis chemistry, there are a huge number of other chemicals present in the plant.

In order to fully understand the medical applications or to produce quality concentrates or marijuana-infused products, a basic understanding of the science is critical. In addition to the better-known cannabinoids THC and CBD, there are dozens of other related cannabinoids found in the plant's cannabis chemistry.

THCA is the natural product version of THC and understanding the chemistry of these two compounds is of utmost importance. Compounds such as CBC and CBG are chemical precursors in the plant biosynthesis of THC and have been shown to have interesting medical properties.

CBN is a degradation product of THC that has unique physiological effects.

Effects

There are different ways of using cannabis, and the method can determine the effects of the drug.

Smoking or inhaling: A sense of elation can start within minutes and peak after 10–30 minutes. The feeling will typically wear off after about 2 hours.

Ingesting: If a person consumes products containing cannabis by mouth, they will usually feel the effects within 1 hour, and the sensations will peak after 2.5–3.5 hours. One study suggests that the type of edible affects the time it takes to feel the effect, with hard candies kicking in quicker.

Topical: Transdermal patches allow the ingredients to enter the body over a prolonged period. This steady infusion can benefit people who are using cannabis to treat pain and inflammation.

What are the effects of secondhand cannabis smoke?

How do cannabinoids work?

The human body naturally produces some cannabinoids through the endocannabinoid system. They act in a similar way to neurotransmitters, sending messages throughout the nervous system.

These neurotransmitters affect brain areas that play a role in memory, thinking, concentration, movement, coordination, sensory and time perception, and pleasure.

The receptors that respond to these cannabinoids also react to THC and other cannabinoids. In this way, cannabinoids from an outside source can change and disrupt normal brain function.

THC appears to affect areas of the brain that control:

memory and attention

balance, posture, and coordination

reaction time

Due to these effects, a person should not drive a car, operate heavy machinery, or engage in risky physical activities after using cannabis.

THC stimulates specific cannabinoid receptors that increase the release of dopamine. Dopamine is a neurotransmitter that relates to feelings of pleasure.

THC can also affect sensory perception. Colors may seem brighter, music more vivid, and emotions more profound.

Do the benefits of cannabis outweigh the risks? Find out here.

What does a person feel?

When people use cannabis, they may notice the following effects:

a feeling of elation or euphoria, known as a high

relaxation

changes in perception, for example, of color, time, and space

an increase in appetite

feeling more talkative

Risks

Using cannabis can also entail some risks. These include:

Impairment of judgment: A 2012 study reported a higher chance of having a road traffic accident when driving within 3 hours of smoking cannabis.

Immune response: A 2019 study showed that frequent cannabis use may affect the immune system, but more studies are necessary to confirm this.

Gum disease: According to the American Dental Association, there may be a link between cannabis use and gum disease

Memory loss: One study found that smokers of potent cannabis strains (skunk, for instance) may have a higher risk of acute memory loss.

Testicular cancer: A 2018 review concluded that using cannabis more than 50 times in a lifetime may increase the risk of testicular cancer.

People have modified some types of cannabis, such as skunk, to maximize the potency of certain components. From the 1990s to 2018, the average THC content in confiscated cannabis rose from 4% to over 15%.

One problem with using unregulated or recreational drugs is that people cannot know exactly what they contain or how strong the effect will be. There may also be contaminants.

Addiction

With long-term use, changes in the brain can occur that lead to problematic use, or cannabis use disorder. This disorder, in which a person experiences withdrawal symptoms when not taking the drug, may affect about 30% of people who use cannabis, according to the National Institute on Drug Abuse (NIDA).

Of these individuals, about 9% may develop an addiction. A person has an addiction when they cannot stop using a substance.

The NIDA add that up to 17% of those who start using cannabis in their teens may become dependent on it.

Cannabis withdrawal

Quitting cannabis, after becoming dependent, is not life threatening, but it can be uncomfortable.

Symptoms may include:

Irritability

mood changes

Insomnia

cravings

restlessness

Decreased appetite

general discomfort

Symptoms tend to peak within the first week after stopping and last up to 2 weeks.

Experts do not know exactly how frequent and long-term cannabis use affects a person's health. Both the short- and long-term effects may vary among individuals.

Can you get high?

Studies have shown that although possible, it is unlikely that a person who breathes in secondhand marijuana smoke will get high.

A high that an otherwise sober person experiences when they are near someone under the influence of recreational drugs is known as a contact high.

The chance of a person becoming high after inhaling secondhand marijuana smoke can increase if they are very close to someone who is smoking. The risk also increases if the person smoking is using marijuana with a higher tetrahydrocannabinol (THC) level.

THC is one of several chemical compounds in the cannabis plant, which are called cannabinoids. It is THC that causes the mind-altering, or psychoactive, effects of weed. Naturally, a higher level of THC means a more potent effect.

If there is poor or no ventilation, the likelihood of a person becoming high from the surrounding smoke drastically increases, too.

In short, for a contact high to be possible, a person would need to be in close contact with highly concentrated marijuana smoke for an extended period in a poorly ventilated area.

Possible side effects

People who inhale secondhand marijuana smoke may feel the following side effects:

burning, itchy, or red eyes

Dry mouth

Headache

coughing

increased appetite

Rapid heartbeat

Anxiety

euphoria

Lightheadedness

A sensation of time slowing

restlessness

Paranoia

tiredness

Nausea

It is also possible that a person who has had exposure to high levels of marijuana smoke in a nonventilated area may experience slight impairments in their memory and motor skills. This effect can be dangerous if a person is driving or operating machinery.

What are the side effects of secondhand marijuana smoke?

Marijuana, the dried leaves and flowers of the cannabis plant, is known for its psychoactive properties. When a person smokes or ingests it, they experience a high. But what about secondhand smoke?

When a person does not smoke marijuana themselves but instead inhales the smoke that someone else breathes out, this is called secondhand marijuana smoking. Some people may be concerned about the risks of breathing this secondhand smoke.

Keep reading to learn more about the effects that secondhand marijuana smoke can have on a person and the possible risks.

Other risks

Exposure to secondhand marijuana smoke carries some other risks, including:

Drug tests

Some workplaces require employees to undergo regular drug tests to make sure that they are drug-free and fit to work. Depending on the sensitivity of the drug test, a positive result may be possible in people who have not directly consumed marijuana but have inhaled secondhand smoke.

In one study, researchers tested urine samples from nonsmokers after they spent an hour in proximity to people smoking marijuana. The researchers found that people who were near to marijuana smokers in poorly ventilated areas did test positive for THC in their urine, based on "commonly utilized cutoff concentrations."

However, the lack of ventilation and strength of the marijuana had a significant effect on the results. Also, the drug tests took place over the period straight after the participants had inhaled the smoke.

Heart health

Although the effects of secondhand cigarette smoke are well-known, experts know little about the associated health risks of secondhand marijuana smoke.

A 2016 study looked into the effects of secondhand marijuana smoke in rats. The researchers found that after a minute of exposure, the femoral artery's response to increased blood flow became impaired for

90 minutes. In comparison, with cigarette smoke, this effect lasted only 30 minutes.

It is possible to conclude from these findings that secondhand marijuana smoke could have negative effects on the heart. However, researchers must continue to study this before making any firm conclusions.

In children

A study into the effect of secondhand marijuana smoke on 83 children with parents who smoke found that almost half of the children had biological evidence of exposure to marijuana.

Although there was no evidence to link secondhand marijuana smoke to health issues in these children, the results are concerning, given the presence of potentially harmful chemicals in marijuana smoke.

Marijuana cigarettes contain various toxins and tars that are also present in tobacco cigarettes, leading researchers to believe that secondhand marijuana smoke possibly carries some of the same health risks as secondhand cigarette smoke. More research is necessary to confirm this, though.

Current studies indicate that secondhand marijuana smoke is unlikely to affect people who experience limited exposure in a well-ventilated environment. However, researchers need to carry out more studies to determine the effects that secondhand marijuana smoke can have on a person.

It is also possible that people with asthma or other breathing issues could be more prone to negative side effects from inhaling secondhand marijuana smoke. However, there is currently no research to support this theory.

In general, contact with secondhand marijuana smoke is unlikely to cause any harmful effects. However, a person who is around people smoking marijuana should be cautious, as there may be unknown risks.

How long can you detect Cannabis in the body?

The length of time this chemical stays in the body or continues to show in a drug test depends on many factors. These include:

How much body fat a person has

How often they consume the drug

How much someone smokes

The sensitivity of the drug test

Drugs such as alcohol may completely disappear from the body in just a few hours. In comparison, weed lingers much longer.

Drug tests can detect tetrahydrocannabinol, or THC, in urine, blood, and hair for many days after use, while saliva tests can only detect THC for a few hours. This is because of the way the body metabolizes THC.

THC is a lipid-soluble chemical. This means that it binds to fat in the body, which increases the length of time it takes for someone to eliminate THC completely.

Cannabis detection windows

Research on the amount of time a test can detect marijuana shows a wide range of averages. Research from 2017 estimates a detection window for a single marijuana cigarette of about 3 days.

The same study emphasizes that detection windows vary and depend on how often a person smokes.

It showed:

For someone smoking marijuana for the first time, tests may detect it for about 3 days.

In someone who smokes marijuana three or four times per week, the detection window is 5–7 days.

For people who smoke marijuana once a day or more, tests may detect it in their system for 30 days or longer.

Detection windows also depend on the kind of test a person undertakes. General estimates for various marijuana tests are as follows:

Urine tests can detect marijuana in the urine for approximately 3–30 days after use.

Saliva tests can detect marijuana for approximately 24 hours after use. Some saliva tests have detected marijuana for up to 72 hours.

Hair tests are the most sensitive tests, detecting THC for up to 90 days after use. However, these tests are testing the oil in skin that transfers to hair, and so they may occasionally show a false positive. A person who comes into contact with a THC user could, theoretically, test positive on a hair test.

Blood tests can only detect THC for 3–4 hours.

How much do you have to smoke to fail a drug test?

Drug tests can detect relatively small quantities of THC, and the amount of THC in a given marijuana cigarette varies. However, little research has examined exactly how much a person must smoke to fail a drug test.

Studies consistently find that frequent weed users are more likely to fail drug tests than infrequent users. A 2012 study in the journal Clinical Chemistry examines marijuana users smoking a single cigarette with 6.8 percent THC.

Urine concentrations of THC were highest 0.6 to 7.4 hours after smoking. Using a highly sensitive urine test, researchers detected THC in the urine of 100 percent of frequent users and 60–100 percent of infrequent users.

A 2017 study reports on testing where hair samples from 136 marijuana users reporting heavy, light, or no use of marijuana. For the study, researchers cut hair into 1-centimeter sections to test for exposure of up to a month prior.

Some 77 percent of heavy users and 39 percent of light users produced positive tests. No non-users had positive test results, suggesting that false positives in hair tests are relatively rare.

Factors that influence detection

Numerous factors influence whether a test detects marijuana, including the following:

Test sensitivity

More sensitive tests can detect lower doses of marijuana. Tests include blood, urine, hair, and saliva.

THC dose

Marijuana drug tests look for THC, not marijuana. So the amount of THC that a person consumes is the significant factor.

The effects of THC are cumulative. This means that a person who smokes several times over several days has consumed a higher THC dose than someone who smokes once, and so they are more likely to test positive.

The strength of each dose of THC also matters. Without sensitive laboratory equipment, a person cannot reliably determine the strength of their marijuana.

How "high" a person feels is also not a reliable measure, because numerous factors other than THC dose can intensify or weaken this feeling.

Body fat

Since fat stores marijuana, people with higher body fat concentrations may metabolize marijuana more slowly than a person with less body fat.

Body mass index (BMI) is one way to judge body fat. However, since weight, and therefore BMI, increase with muscle mass, BMI is not a perfect measure of body fat.

Sex

Typically, females have more body fat than males. This means that females may metabolize marijuana slightly more slowly.

Hydration

Dehydration increases concentrations of THC in the body. While drinking lots of water is unlikely to affect a drug test significantly, severe dehydration might.

Exercise

Exercise will not significantly change the rate at which the body metabolizes THC. Exercising before a drug test, however, might.

A small study of 14 regular marijuana users assesses the effects of 35 minutes of exercise on a stationary bike. The results conclude that THC concentrations increased by a statistically significant amount, suggesting that exercise right before a drug test may increase the likelihood of a positive test result.

The researchers believe that exercise may cause fat cells to release THC. In their results, people with higher BMI had more significant increases in THC levels.

Metabolism

For a drug test to be negative, the body must eliminate THC from the system, as well as metabolic chemicals that have links to THC. People with faster metabolisms typically eliminate THC more quickly than those with slower metabolisms.

How to get Cannabis out of the body faster

Ultimately, there are only two strategies that work for this, and they are decreasing the concentration of THC in the marijuana and speeding up the metabolism.

Proper hydration can prevent a drug test from showing unusually high THC concentrations. For people whose test results are on the border of positive and negative, this means that being dehydrated may increase the chances of a positive result.

There is no reliable way to speed up the metabolism. Exercise might help the body metabolize more THC, but exercising too near to a test may also cause a positive result.

The single most important factor is the time from the last exposure to the time of testing.

There is no way to accurately predict the amount of time it will take an individual to metabolize marijuana and eliminate it from their bodies. Home tests can help people test themselves for the presence of marijuana in their system.

For almost all people, marijuana should disappear or be very low in concentration within 30 days. For infrequent users, it may take 10 days or less for marijuana to leave the body.

What does it feel like to be high on cannabis?

For years, people have associated cannabis with recreational use and "getting high." Though many people may talk about the effects of cannabis, it is important to understand that different people may have very varied reactions to cannabis use.

According to the National Institute on Drug Abuse, cannabis is the "most commonly used illicit drug" in the United States. In fact, a 2015 drug abuse and use survey stated that over 22 million people used cannabis in a single month.

Keep reading for more information on what it feels like to be high on cannabis, what causes it, and the factors that can affect how a person may respond to cannabis in its various forms.

Cannabis contains hundreds of compounds. Scientists and researchers are particularly interested in two of these chemical compounds: cannabidiol (CBD) and delta-9-tetrahydrocannabinol (THC).

THC produces the high when a person smokes, ingests, or vapes it. It enters the bloodstream and makes its way to the brain. It then attaches to receptors in the brain, which causes the high to occur in most people.

THC also slows down communication between the brain and rest of the body, which gives cannabis its calming effect.

Proponents of recreational cannabis use often talk about the positive effects of being high. These sensations can include:

A feeling of relaxation

Euphoria

Laughter or giggles

Hunger

Greater amusement and enjoyment

Greater sensitivity to color, touch, smell, light, taste, and sound

A feeling of being more creative

Cannabis can cause the body to become dependent on the good feelings it produces.

Over time, a person's body may greatly reduce the number of endocrines it creates because the chemicals within cannabis replace the naturally occurring chemicals present in the body. However, this is still just a theory, as there has been no research yet.

The stages of being high

THC levels in the blood vary over time. Generally, they will build until they peak, and once they peak, they start to work their way out of the blood through a person's urine or stool.

As THC levels rise and fall, a person may experience different effects from cannabis. During the peak, a person is most likely to experience the euphoric effect. As the THC concentrations in the blood begin to fall, however, a person may experience:

Hunger

Sleepiness

Anxiety or mild paranoia

The speed at which a person goes through these stages, and which stages they experience, will depend on several factors, including:

The method of use, such as vaping, smoking, or ingesting

Strain

Potency

Dose

Sex

Age

Physiology

Frequency of use

Use of alcohol or other drugs while using cannabis.

Strains

The term "strain" refers to the subspecies of the cannabis plant. There are three main strains of cannabis: Cannabis indica, Cannabis sativa, and a hybrid of the two.

In general, frequent users of cannabis believe that Cannabis indica strains produce a sensation of relaxation, while Cannabis sativa strains produce more of the euphoric high, which is better for creativity and social interaction. A hybrid strain may cause both effects, to varying degrees.

However, according to an interview with Dr. Ethan Russo, an established expert on the human endocannabinoid system, there is no evidence to suggest that the different strains actually produce different effects.

Instead, he explained that the differences are based on how a person reacts to the individual plant and the amount of terpenoids within the particular plant the person is using. More research is needed in this area, however.

Methods of consumption

There are several different ways of using cannabis. The three most common methods of use are:

Smoking

Vaping

Using edibles, such as brownies or candies

THC absorption differs depending on the method a person uses. For example, when a person smokes or vapes cannabis, the effects of being high occur almost immediately. The THC enters the lungs and bloodstream, and the user very quickly reaches their peak high.

When a person ingests cannabis in the form of edibles, however, it has to travel through the digestive tract, which slows down the process of absorption into the blood. Therefore, it takes longer for the effects of the edibles to kick in. Take care not to take too much while waiting for an effect.

In 2016, a review of studies identified the following time frames for smoking, vaping, and using edibles:

Smoking or vaping Edibles

Onset Within a few minutes 30–90 minutes

Peak 20–30 minutes 3 hours

Total time 2–3 hours around 24 hours

CBD vs. THC

CBD and THC are two of many different compounds present in cannabis. CBD and THC both interact with cannabinoid receptors, but only THC causes the high that people associate with recreational cannabis use. Learn more about the similarities and differences here.

CBD does not cause a high. Manufacturers often extract CBD from the cannabis plant for medicinal use. Healthcare professionals have used CBD to treat pain, anxiety, and several other medical conditions.

THC is present in the bud of the cannabis plant, which is why people tend to use these parts in recreational joints and edibles.

Possible side effects of being very high

If a person smokes, vapes, or consumes too much cannabis, they may experience unpleasant effects. These might include:

Panic

Psychosis

Confusion

Anxiety

Paranoia

delusions

Hallucinations

nausea and vomiting

red eyes

delayed reaction times

reduced muscle and limb coordination

increased heart rate

distorted senses

People who do not use cannabis regularly are more likely to experience these unpleasant effects from being high.

It is unclear whether or not there are long-term side effects of using cannabis. Researchers must determine what, if any, long-term complications of cannabis use exist.

Generally, there are minimal side effects when using cannabis to get high. According to Americans for Safe Access, a person would need to smoke the equivalent of 1,500 pounds of cannabis in 15 minutes to overdose. However, this is untested and more or less impossible.

The National Institute of Drug Abuse warn that a person who has used too much cannabis may experience acute psychosis, the effects of which can include hallucinations, delusions, and loss of personal identity.

A person is also more likely to become very high on cannabis if they use edibles. This is because when a person consumes edibles, the cannabis has to pass through the digestive system before it enters the bloodstream.

The result of this is a delay of the onset of the high associated with cannabis. This delay can cause a person to eat more than needed as they wait for the effects to kick in.

The American Addiction Centers also warn that some people who deal cannabis may mix it with additional drugs. They cite the following potential side effects:

Hyperactivity or aggressiveness

Cardiac arrest

Stroke

Seizures

High blood pressure

Headache

Chest pain

Hyperactivity

Aggressive behavior

Irregular heartbeat

It is important to note that these additional side effects would be the result of the drugs added to the cannabis. Pure cannabis should not cause these more severe side effects.

Cannabis extracts are a growing segment of the cannabis market as consumers begin to discover their versatility and health benefits when compared to traditional forms of cannabis consumption.

What is Cannabis Extract?

Cannabis extracts entail a wide category of products that includes any extract of the cannabis plant, including extracts from marijuana and hemp. These extracts contain high levels of cannabinoids like CBD and THC, much higher by weight than the dry cannabis flowers, leaves, or stems. Hemp extracts will contain higher levels of CBD, while marijuana extracts have higher levels of THC. The high concentrations of cannabinoids in cannabis extracts mean that you can vape less and less often than if you were to smoke dry flowers.

Cannabis extracts are created by passing a solvent through finely ground cured or fresh cannabis material, including the flower, leaves, and stems. When made with fresh flowers, extracts are sometimes called live resin. Common solvents include safe choices like CO_2 or solvents like butane, hexane, and more that can be toxic if not properly purged from the extract.

Marijuana extracts can also be made by hot pressing fresh or dry marijuana buds, allowing the flower's oil to squeeze out. When created this way, extracts are called rosin.

It is possible to buy pressed rosin commercially, but home rosin pressing kits have made rosin a common DIY cannabis extract. All that is needed to make rosin is heat and pressure, so it can even be crafted with no more than parchment paper and a flat iron.

Once extracted, cannabis oil can be processed into a number of different forms, like shatter, budder, wax, vape liquid, sap, and more. It can even be filtered down to isolate the cannabinoids, creating incredibly pure THC or CBD crystals.

Because of the various forms they can take, cannabis extracts are versatile enough to be used in ways like vaping, dabbing, making edibles, and boosting the potency of cannabis flower in joints or pipes.

Vaporizing

Vaping is a trending way to use cannabis extracts due to the portability and discrete nature of most cannabis extract vapes. The ability to vape cannabis on your own terms is a big selling point for vapes over other forms of consumption.

Vaping cannabis extracts works by heating the extract to its vaporization point, releasing cannabinoid loaded vapor that you can inhale. Cannabinoids and other active compounds are rapidly absorbed through the lungs and into the bloodstream.

The heating element in a vaporizer is typically called the atomizer. When exposed to the atomizer, cannabis extracts are heated to vaporization, creating vapor, but not smoke.

The most common vaporizers for cannabis extracts are vape pens. These highly portable vaporizers combine rechargeable batteries with a heating element and mouthpiece for a discreet, easy to use way to enjoy cannabis extracts.

Some vape pens are designed to be used with cannabis extracts like shatter, wax, sap, isolate, and similar extract forms.

Other vape pens are made to use a vape liquid or oil. These pens sometimes come with refillable cartridges or "tanks". These refillable cartridges can be filled with cannabis extract infused liquids like CBD Vape Liquid from Dixie Botanicals. You can get started vaping CBD with our CBD Vape Starter Bundles.

It is also possible to purchase prefilled, disposable vape cartridges that fit most 510 threaded batteries. These prefilled cartridges are available in both THC and CBD infused vape oils. THC vapes can be purchased at your local medical or recreational marijuana dispensary if you live in a state where marijuana has been legalized. CBD vape cartridges from Dixie Botanicals made from hemp are available now for purchase in the Medical Marijuana, Inc. Store.

Everything you need to know about ways to consume cannabis extracts like oil, shatter, budder, sap, and isolate.

Cannabis extracts are a growing segment of the cannabis market as consumers begin to discover their versatility and health benefits when compared to traditional forms of cannabis consumption.

Here, we look at the different ways you can use your cannabis extracts, but first, let's learn a bit more about what cannabis extracts are and how they are made.

What Are Extracts?

Extracts (also known as concentrates) is actually an umbrella term for the variety of products that can be produced when cannabis flower is processed into a concentrated form. These products can come in liquid or solid form, such as cannabis oil, hash, vape cartridge liquid, shatter, wax, kief, tinctures, and are either ingested or inhaled.

The process for creating extracts varies depending on the intended finished product, but the basic goal is to isolate and remove the cannabinoids and terpenes. During the concentration process, dried or fresh cannabis plants can be sifted; exposed to heat or extreme cold, gas (such as carbon dioxide), a solvent, another oil or a combination of these; or further refined using ethanol.

Cannabis extracts are created by passing a solvent through finely ground cured or fresh cannabis material, including the flower, leaves, and stems. When made with fresh flowers, extracts are sometimes called live resin. Common solvents include safe choices like CO_2 or solvents like butane, hexane, and more that can be toxic if not properly purged from the extract.

Marijuana extracts can also be made by hot pressing fresh or dry marijuana buds, allowing the flower's oil to squeeze out.

When created this way, extracts are called rosin.

It is possible to buy pressed rosin commercially, but home rosin pressing kits have made rosin a common DIY cannabis extract. All that is needed to make rosin is heat and pressure, so it can even be crafted with no more than parchment paper and a flat iron.

Once extracted, cannabis oil can be processed into a number of different forms, like shatter, budder, wax, vape liquid, sap, and more. It can even be filtered down to isolate the cannabinoids, creating incredibly pure THC or CBD crystals.

Because of the various forms they can take, cannabis extracts are versatile enough to be used in ways like vaping, dabbing, making edibles, and boosting the potency of cannabis flower in joints or pipes.

How Do They Work?

The way the cannabinoids in the cannabis extract enter your body depends on the form of extract and method of consumption. When cannabis extract is ingested, it can produce effects that are similar to those experienced when cannabis flower is smoked or vaped; however the effects may be delayed due to digestion, which can take from 30 minutes up to four hours or more. When cannabis extracts are inhaled (such as by dabbing or vaping), the tetrahydrocannabinol, or THC, is absorbed by the blood in the lungs and moves quickly to the brain, producing an almost immediate effect, possibly within minutes.

The duration of potential effects also depend on how the cannabis extract is consumed. If it's inhaled, effects can last one to three hours, or longer. When extract is ingested, effects can be felt for up to 12 hours. The timing of the onset and duration of effects vary from person to person. Individual factors such as sex, mental and physical health, age, personality, genetics and even the amount of food ingested prior to consumption all play a part.

How Are Extracts Different from Other Types of Cannabis?

The main difference between extracts and other forms of cannabis is in their potential to contain much higher concentrations of cannabinoids than the raw plant. For example, extracts can have up to 90% THC, while dried flower typically contains 1% to 30% THC. Extracts available through OCS that are meant to be inhaled can contain no more than 1,000 mg of THC per package; ingestible extracts contain no more than 10 mg of THC per unit.

What Are the Pros and Cons of Consuming Extracts?

Depending on their form, extracts can be a smoke-free alternative to inhaling cannabis, which may come with risks to lung health. The higher concentration of THC may increase the risk of overconsumption.

Vaporizing

Vaping is a trending way to use cannabis extracts due to the portability and discrete nature of most cannabis extract vapes. The ability to vape cannabis on your own terms is a big selling point for vapes over other forms of consumption.

Vaping cannabis extracts works by heating the extract to its vaporization point, releasing cannabinoid loaded vapor that you can inhale. Cannabinoids and other active compounds are rapidly absorbed through the lungs and into the bloodstream.

The heating element in a vaporizer is typically called the atomizer. When exposed to the atomizer, cannabis extracts are heated to vaporization, creating vapor, but not smoke.

The most common vaporizers for cannabis extracts are vape pens. These highly portable vaporizers combine rechargeable batteries with a heating element and mouthpiece for a discreet, easy to use way to enjoy cannabis extracts.

Some vape pens are designed to be used with cannabis extracts like shatter, wax, sap, isolate, and similar extract forms. You can learn more about vaping wax or shatter like marijuana extracts here.

Other vape pens are made to use a vape liquid or oil. These pens sometimes come with refillable cartridges or "tanks". These refillable cartridges can be filled with cannabis extract infused liquids like CBD Vape Liquid from Dixie Botanicals®. You can get started vaping CBD with our CBD Vape Starter Bundles.

It is also possible to purchase prefilled, disposable vape cartridges that fit most 510 threaded batteries. These prefilled cartridges are available in both THC and CBD infused vape oils. THC vapes can be purchased at your local medical or recreational marijuana dispensary if you live in a state where marijuana has been legalized. CBD vape cartridges from Dixie Botanicals® made from hemp are available now for purchase in the Medical Marijuana, Inc. store.

Dabbing

Another way to enjoy cannabis extracts is by dabbing them. Dabbing is a form of vaporizing and works on much the same principle as vape pens in that the extract is applied to a heating element in order to cause its vaporization.

Dabbing is traditionally more popular among more experienced cannabis consumers because it requires a set of specialized hardware to get started. However, anyone can take advantage of the benefits of dabbing, including robust, flavorful vapor and an increased potency that means you can consume less and do so less often.

In order to get started dabbing, you'll need a few tools, including a torch similar to those used to make creme brulee, a specially equipped water pipe called a dab rig, and a surface that can be heated like a titanium or ceramic nail or a quartz bucket.

To dab your extract, you will first fill your water pipe until the downstem is cover with water. Next, load your dab onto your dab tool. Remember, you won't need much. It is best to start small until you know how you will be affected. Then, using your torch, you'll heat your nail or bucket until it just starts to glow red. Allow it to cool for a few seconds, then carefully dab your extract on the hot surface while inhaling from the dab rig's mouthpiece.

Although dabbing is usually done with high-THC marijuana extracts, more and more consumers are beginning to dab CBD extracts derived from hemp for their CBD content.

Dabbing Without a Rig

Even as dabbing spreads in popularity as a way to vaporize botanical extracts, it is earning a stigma for its use of flame to heat the dabbing surface, scaring off some potential users.

Enter the Dr. Dabber Switch Vaporizer – this unique cordless e-rig gives consumers the chance to dab without the flame and red hot surfaces tied to dabbing.

Instead of using a torch to heat a nail or bucket, the Switch from Dr. Dabber uses its powerful battery to heat your botanical extracts to their vaporization point using induction heating, creating potent clouds of vapor.

With its percolator attachment, the Dr. Dabber Switch utilizes the same water function as dab rigs to cool and clean your vapor, making it as close to a dab as you can get with an electronic vape.

As a bonus, the Dr. Dabber Switch can also vaporize your favorite dry botanicals, making it a versatile choice in vaporizer.

Can You Dab with a Vape Pen?

Dabbing is just a way to flash vaporize your botanical extracts using a heat source. Using that definition, vape pens designed to vape botanicals concentrates give you the ability to easily and discreetly "dab" on the go.

A vape pen uses its battery to power its atomizer or heating element, often coils around a cotton or ceramic wick. Your waxy concentrate will be heated to its vaporization point by the atomizer, releasing a vapor that can be inhaled off of the vape's mouthpiece.

To vape your waxy concentrates, you will open your vape pen to access the chamber where you add your extract. Using the tool likely included with your vape, you will load your extract into your vape pen according to its users manual, being careful not to overfill.

Once your extract is loaded, you are ready to vape. Press your vape's button and inhale or, if it is autodraw, just take a puff from your vape's mouthpiece to activate it.

Choosing a Wax Vape

Vape pens that are capable of vaporizing botanical extracts like wax come in a variety of sizes and price points. Some vapes come with features like adjustable heat settings; others give you the ability to vaporize a variety of extracts and even dry herb.

Adding to Cannabis Flower

Some consumers use cannabis extracts to boost the CBD or THC potency of their favorite cannabis flower or other smokable dry herbs. This can be done in a couple ways.

First, cannabis extracts can be added on top of marijuana flower in a pipe before smoking. When lighting a bowl that has been topped with cannabis extract, be careful, as it may flare up, creating a large flame. Instead, hold your flame just above your pipe's bowl as you inhale. This will partially vaporize the extract. The rest may melt, coating your flower. Use care as you finish smoking your pipe, as the extract may continue to increase the flammability of your flower.

It is also possible to add cannabis extract to a joint or blunt. Some users will add their marijuana concentrate to their marijuana flower or other dry herb as they roll their joint or blunt. This works best if you have a messy extract like oil or a crumbly extract like honeycomb and isolates. It is also possible to add cannabis extract to the outside of a joint or blunt, sometimes called twaxing.

This method works best when you have a sticky extract like shatter or sap that will hold to the paper of your joint or blunt. Like when you add cannabis extract to your pipe, adding it to a joint or blunt may cause it to flare up or burn unevenly, so take care when using this method.

Infusing Edibles

Cannabis extracts can also be used to infuse foods and beverages with cannabinoids like THC or CBD.

Because cannabinoids degrade when exposed to high heat, it is not recommended that you cook with cannabis extracts using temperatures above 375 degrees F. However, with vaporization points as low as 315 degrees F, some loss of potency can still occur when cooking with cannabis extracts.

For that reason, it is often suggested that cannabis extracts be added to foods and beverages after they are cooked. This will reduce exposure of cannabinoids to high heat and minimize loss of potency.

Remember that it is best to use cannabis extracts that have been decarboxylated if you are looking to consume CBD or THC, rather than their non-carboxylated forms CBDa and THCa. This is especially important when using extracts with THC since THCa is non-psychoactive.

Powdered THC or CBD isolate powder are exceptionally suited for infusing cannabinoids into your favorite foods or beverages because they can be sprinkled and mixed into foods without separation.

Conclusion

Just before you purchase a cannabis extract, read the label or the information available on the product page at OCS.ca so you know how much THC and CBD it contains. If you are trying extracts for the first time, choose a product with a low level of THC or a high amount of CBD, which can counter the unpleasant effects of THC.